YOUR KNOWLEDGE HAS VALUE

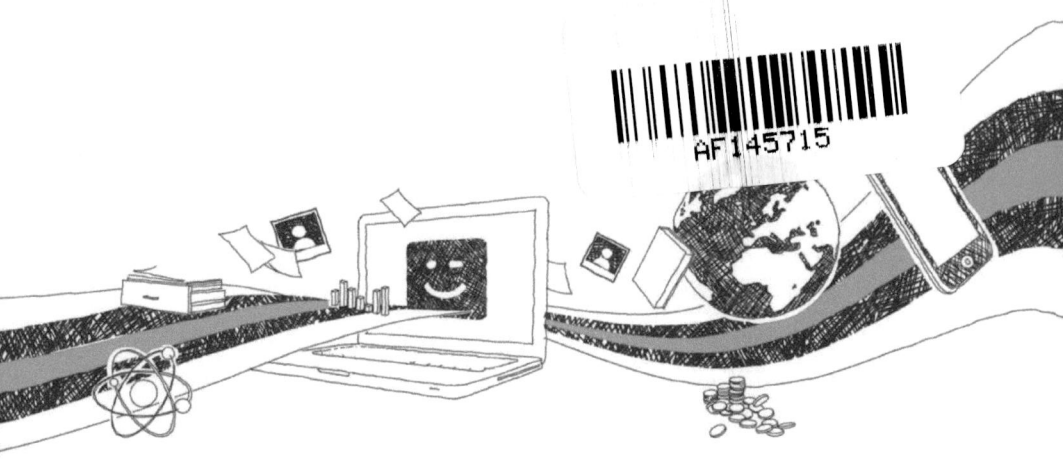

AF145715

- We will publish your bachelor's and master's thesis, essays and papers

- Your own eBook and book - sold worldwide in all relevant shops

- Earn money with each sale

Upload your text at www.GRIN.com and publish for free

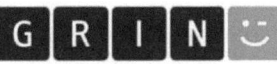

Bibliographic information published by the German National Library:

The German National Library lists this publication in the National Bibliography; detailed bibliographic data are available on the Internet at http://dnb.dnb.de .

Imprint:

Copyright © 2014 GRIN Verlag, Open Publishing GmbH
Print and binding: Books on Demand GmbH, Norderstedt Germany
ISBN: 9783668390515

This book at GRIN:

http://www.grin.com/en/e-book/352611/the-different-mechanisms-through-which-immune-tolerance-to-antigens-can

Charlotte Leahy

The different mechanisms through which immune tolerance to antigens can occur, and their relative importance in preventing the development of allergic disease

GRIN Publishing

GRIN - Your knowledge has value

Since its foundation in 1998, GRIN has specialized in publishing academic texts by students, college teachers and other academics as e-book and printed book. The website www.grin.com is an ideal platform for presenting term papers, final papers, scientific essays, dissertations and specialist books.

Visit us on the internet:

http://www.grin.com/

http://www.facebook.com/grincom

http://www.twitter.com/grin_com

Table of Contents

Allergy 2

Central Tolerance 3

    T-cell tolerance 4

    B-cell Tolerance 5

Peripheral Tolerance 6

    Anergy 6

    Deletion 7

    B cell antibody production 8

Immune Deviation 10

Regulatory Lymphocytes 11

    Regulatory T cells: Treg, Tr1, Th3 11

    Regulatory B cells: Breg, Br1, Br3 13

Innate Immune System: Dendritic cells 14

Immune Privilege 18

Tolerance in Pregnancy 18

Induced Tolerance 18

Conclusion 19

References 20

The different mechanisms through which immune tolerance to antigens can occur, and their relative importance in preventing the development of allergic disease

Leahy, C 2014

Immune tolerance is the inhibition or absence of an immune response leaving only protective and beneficial immunity intact. Tolerance reduces response to both self and non-self antigens, which are substances which stimulate antibody production.

Tolerance breakdown causes immune disease; failed self-tolerance causes incorrect identification of self as foreign, causing autoimmune disease[1]. Failure of induced tolerance causes overzealous identification of harmless foreign substances as a threat, causing hypersensitivities[2].

Allergy

Allergy occurs when a harmful immune response develops to an otherwise harmless foreign substance (the 'allergen'); mainly type I hypersensitivity, although it can be mixed with type IV[3]. Type I is immediate hypersensitivity reaction, mediated by IgE. Antigens are presented to specific Th2 cells that release IL-4 and IL-13, stimulating B cell production of antigen-specific IgE. The atopic immune system has a polarised Th2 population[4].

Initial exposure causes sensitisation and allergen-specific IgE formation. During acute reactions, mediators such as prostaglandins and histamine are released by mast cells (figure 1) leading to allergy symptoms.

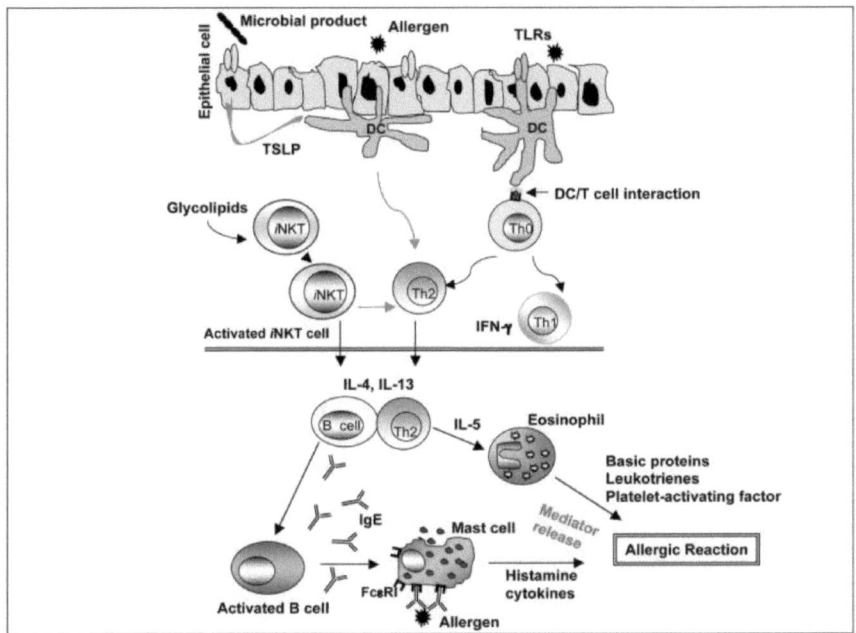

Figure 1: Mechanism of tolerance taken from Li et al 2008[4]

After dendritic cells (DCs) encounter the allergen they promote Th2 cell proliferation. Th2 cells produce IL-4 and IL-13. These cytokines help switch mature B cell to IgE isotype. IgE binds to FcɛR1 on mast cells and cross-links them causing degranulation of allergy mediators. Allergic asthma pulmonary iNKT cells are activated by glycolipid antigens and can amplify Th2 response. Eosinophils also contribute to allergic response, particularly in the lungs.

Type IV delayed type hypersensitivity (DTH) is cell-mediated chronic inflammation driven by macrophage IL-12 and allergen-specific T cell IFN-γ cross-talk and TNF release[3]. It is often a skin reaction, eg to nickel, driven by Th1 cells inducing tissue cell apoptosis.

<u>Central Tolerance</u>

Central tolerance, first theorised in 1959 by Joshua Lederberg[5], is the induction of lymphocyte apoptosis or anergy within primary lymphoid organs; bone marrow for B cells and the thymus for T cells. It prevents self-reactive lymphocytes entering the circulation.

T-cell tolerance

T-cells respond to antigens in the context of major histocompatibility complex (MHC) on antigen presenting cells (APCs). Activation requires co-stimulation of both the cell-surface T cell receptor (TCR) and CD28 by the MHC and B7 on the APC, with lack of co-stimulatory CD28 engagement causing anergy[6].

Within the thymus, cells are retained or excluded according to their receptor affinity for peptide antigen, leaving a pool of functionally useful T-cells (figure 2), with ~98% dying during selection[7]. Firstly, pluripotent haemopoietic stem cells from the bone marrow produce precursor CD4⁻CD8⁻T-cells which seed in the thymus from week eight of development[8]. β-repertoire selection ensures thymocytes with a functional TCR β-chain survive and divide, with TCRα gene rearrangement and differentiation to $CD4^+CD8^+$ $αβ^+$ cells.

Positive selection of thymocytes which have self-MHC binding, during MHC presentation by thymic DCs, occurs and thymocytes which fail die 'by neglect'. Negative selection occurs during overly strong responses to MHC, resulting in apoptosis, ensuring self tolerance.

Autoimmune regulator (AIRE) is a transcriptional control element which promotes central tolerance during negative selection by enhancing antigen-presentation by thymic DCs[9]. When AIRE is absent autoimmunity overwhelms the body.

The resulting mature cells are either $CD4^+$ in response to MHC class II or $CD8^+$ to MHC class I. Thymic DCs also drive regulatory T cell formation, which has a large role in peripheral tolerance.

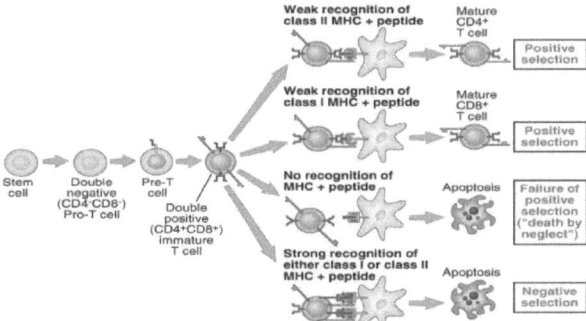

Figure 2: Mechanisms of central tolerance of T cells in the thymus, taken from Takahama et al, 2006[7]

Positive selection to ensures survival of CD4+ and CD8+ T cells capable of recognising MHC classes. Negative selection prevents unwanted strong immune response to the body's own tissues and prevents autoimmunity. "Death by neglect" is where positive selection has failed due the no recognition of MHC and peptide.

B-cell Tolerance

B cells are part of the humoral immune response, primarily making antibodies against specific antigens. In the context of allergy they are stimulated by Th2 cells producing IL-4 to switch immunoglobulin classes to IgE.

During the transitional phase in B cell maturity, induction of tolerance occurs that helps shape the final B cell receptor (BCR) repertoire. Immature B cells encounter self antigens in the bone marrow and negative selection ensures that the cells which are self-reactive undergo apoptosis or anergy[9]. Where BCR has limited cross-linking to self-antigens, anergy occurs. Where multivalent self-antigens cause extensive BCR cross-linking the B cell undergoes maturational arrest and receptor editing. Unsuccessful receptor revision leads to cell apoptosis and successful revision results in a pool of mature B cells which are not self-reactive.

Whilst central tolerance is vital for preventing autoimmune disease and some hypersensitivities it does not have an obvious role allergy, other than the production of regulatory T cells (Tregs).

Peripheral Tolerance

Central tolerance is not foolproof and antigens from peripheral tissues do not circulate within the primary lymphoid tissues. This can lead auto-reactive lymphocytes circulating in the body, with T cells and B cells being modulated or deleted to ensure no auto-reactivity and to suppress response to harmless external antigens.

Peripheral tolerance of T cells is regulated by intrinsic and extrinsic mechanisms. Intrinsic mechanisms involve T cell anergy, phenotype skewing and deletion and extrinsic mechanisms involve regulatory T cells, cytokines and APCs. Impairment of these mechanisms can lead to allergy.

Anergy

T cell anergy is induced by antigen recognition leading to functional inactivation, where the cell remains alive in a hyporesponsive state[10]. There are two types of anergy; clonal anergy and adaptive tolerance (table 1).

Clonal anergy arises from incomplete T cell activation, inhibiting cell cycle progression and IL-2 secretion. Anergy can be broken by exogenous IL-2[11]. It is induced in CD4+ T cells about 6–12 h after strong TCR signal in the absence of costimulation, or by a low-affinity ligand with inhibitory costimulation, blocking the Ras/MAP kinase pathway with indirect blockage of the cell cycle and inhibiting IL-2 production[12]. The CD28/B7 costimulation is vital in blocking anergy, although other costimulation pathways have roles, such as ICAM-1/LFA-1[13].

Adaptive tolerance anergy occurs when cells down-regulate proliferation and differentiation functions due to persistent antigens and can be reversed in antigen absence[10]. It involves a block in tyrosine kinase activation and IL-2 receptor signalling. Both anergic states can be found in Tregs, preventing them from dominating and suppressing immune responses prematurely. B cell suppression is another mechanism by which inflammatory response is reduced[14].

Table 1: Comparing clonal anergy and adaptive tolerance in T cells

Characteristic	Clonal anergy	Adaptive tolerance
Cell type affected	Activated CD4+/CD8+	Naive CD4+/CD8+
Antigen persistence necessary	No	Yes
Proliferation inhibition	Yes	Yes
CTLA-4	No	Yes
Inhibition of cytokines	IL-2	IL-2, IFNγ, IL-4
Signalling pathway blocked	Ras/MAP kinase	Ca/Tyr kinase
Reversible	Yes (by IL-2 or anti-Ox40)	Yes (by Anti-Ox40)

Allergy may be secondary to impaired anergy of lymphocytes as shown by Macaubus et al[15]. They showed that in normal individuals allergen-specific T cells are present at lower levels and have different proliferation requirements to those in allergic individuals due to anergy.

Deletion

Unlike central deletion, peripheral deletion involves activation-induced apoptosis. Deletion can occur in B and Th1/2 cells. When chronically responding to peptide-MHC complexes a combination of events occur to induce apoptosis: Fas receptor is engaged by FasL, Bim-dependent triggering of a Bcl-2 and Bcl-xL–regulated mitochondrial death pathway[16]. It is used in oral tolerance to prevent food allergy where antigen-reactive T cells in Peyer's patches are deleted.[17]

B cell antibody production

Antibody class is determined by the heavy chain constant (C_H) region which is bound by Fc receptors on the cell surface. Class switching occurs in mature B cells in response to antigen stimulation and costimulation by CD40 and toll-like receptors or cytokines, eg IL-4, from T cells or DCs. This causes an intrachromosomal deletional recombination event (figure 3) within switch regions located upstream of the CH region genes[18]. Naïve mature B cells initially express IgM and IgD, and can switch to IgG, IgA and IgE sequentially- with the inability to switch back from IgE. IgE mediates allergic response, with antibody classes such as IgG4 and IgA regarded as being tolorogenic[19].

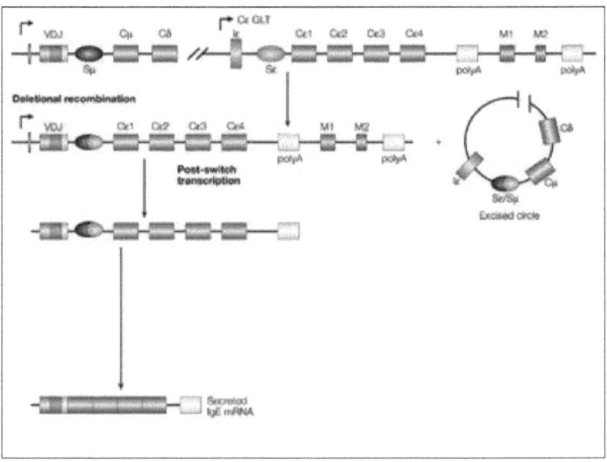

Figure 3: Class switching of isotypes in B cells to IgE antibody type. Modified from Geha et al, 2003[22]

B cells produce IgM antibodies, with production of other isotypes having the same specificity requiring heavy chain alteration. A large piece of genomic DNA from μ switch (Sμ) to Sε is excised and the VJD is ligated to the Sε sequence.

Cytokines are mediators of immune response which can induce immunity or tolerance. In allergy the Th2 cytokines (including IL-4, IL-13 and IL-5) and Th1 IFNγ induce the systemic reaction[20]. Immune deviation is affected by circulating cytokines with IL-4 inducing Th2 and IL-12 inducing Th1 differentiation[21].

IL-10 and TGF-β are generally regarded as important in tolerance and allergy prevention (table 2) due to their anti-inflammatory properties and ability to down-regulated antigen-specific response in T cells[22]. They are produced by many cell types, including Tregs, Th1 cells and B cells.

Table 2: Comparing the functions of IL-10 and TGF-β in the prevention of allergy[22-24]

IL-10	TGF-β
Decreases allergen-specific IgE	Decreases allergen-specific IgE
Increases allergen-specific IgG4	Increases allergen-specific IgA
Induces T cells anergy	Suppresses T cell proliferation
Inhibits DC maturation	Decrease DC response to IgE
Increases Treg response	Increases Treg response
Inhibits allergy-mediator release	Blocks T cells costimulatory mechanisms

Peripheral tolerance of T cells depends on signalling via co-stimulatory molecules. Members of the CD28 family are particularly important, such as cytotoxic T-lymphocyte antigen-4 (CTLA-4) and programmed death-1 (PD-1)[25].

CTLA-4 is expressed in T cell activation with the ability block CD28 activation and to halt cell-cycle progression[26]. In knockout mice there is increased T cell proliferation and autoimmune disease[27]. PD-1 seems to maintain tolerance and anergy[28]. These molecules can act synergistically to induce tolerance, as seen in DC regulation of cytotoxic cells[29]. In allergy this mechanism has not been well defined, although it is used by Tr1 cells[30].

Immune Deviation

Lymphocytes can differentiate towards antigen-specific cells with different functions and cytokine spectrums. T cell populations can have a Th2 or Th1 phenotype[21]. After antigen activation, CD4+ T cell precursors differentiate into either Th1 cells, which activate macrophages and mediating DTH, or Th2 cells which predispose to atopy, cause antibody responses and mediate allergic reactions[20].

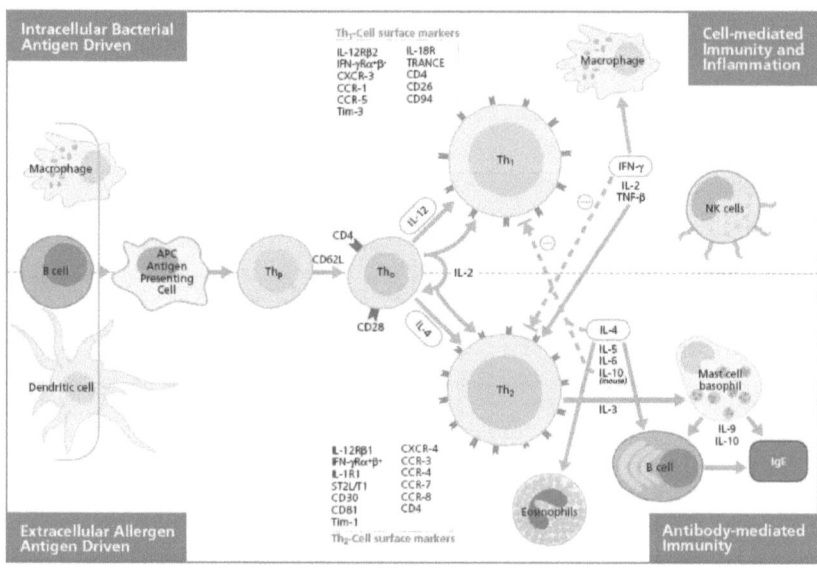

Figure 4: Relationship between immune deviation, Th2 immune response and allergy

Presentation of an antigen to a naïve T cell causes it to mature into an effector T cell, with polarization affected by circulating cytokines. Th1 produce IFNγ, IL-2, IL-10 and TNFβ and Th2 produce IL-4, IL-5 and IL-13.

Th2 exerts its effect by stimulating B cell antibody mediated immunity, with IgE responsible for the manifestation of acute allergic response. Th1 and Th2 cells have cross-talk through cytokines such as IFNγ and IL-2

In healthy individuals deviation is controlled by cytokine cross-over and by Tregs. Th2 cell suppression reduces cytokines which activate allergy cells (eg mast cells) and B cell class-switching to IgE.

The hygiene hypothesis suggests that early exposure to microbes shifts allergen-specific response from Th2 to Th1 phenotype, via Tregs and innate immunity modulation[4] and evidence suggests prenatal exposure influences later phenotype too[31].

Regulatory Lymphocytes

Regulatory T cells: Treg, Tr1, Th3

Tregs and their regulatory cytokines (eg IL-10, TGF-β) contribute to maintaining immune tolerance[22].

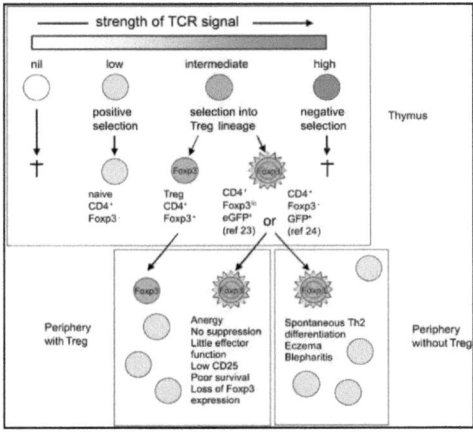

Figure 7: Thymic selection of natural Treg cells and its consequence for peripheral regulation, taken from Fazekas et al, 2007[35]

The avidity of Treg cells for self-antigen can lead to negative selection when high and positive selection when low. When they are Foxp3- their differentiation is subverted.

Tregs are derived from the thymus as CD4+CD25+Foxp3+T cells. Foxp3 is the main transcription factor; lack of Foxp3 causes IPEX syndrome, a lymphoproliferative disease with autoimmune and allergic characteristics such as hyper-IgE syndrome, allergic airway and eosinophilia[32], showing Treg importance in preventing allergy.

Tregs modulate immune tolerance through regulating many cell types (figure 8). They alter APC function through CTLA4-B7 interactions, bind and endocytose B7 molecules (blocking antigen presentation) and increase pro-apoptotic metabolites by lymphocyte-activation gene 3 binding to MHC class II, inhibiting APC maturation and function[24]. They also promote IL-10 producing DCs.

Tregs cause T cell suppression by cytolytic mechanisms; binding cells and secreting granzymes[33]. Cell surface galectin-1 and suppressor-cytokines cause cell-cycle arrest.

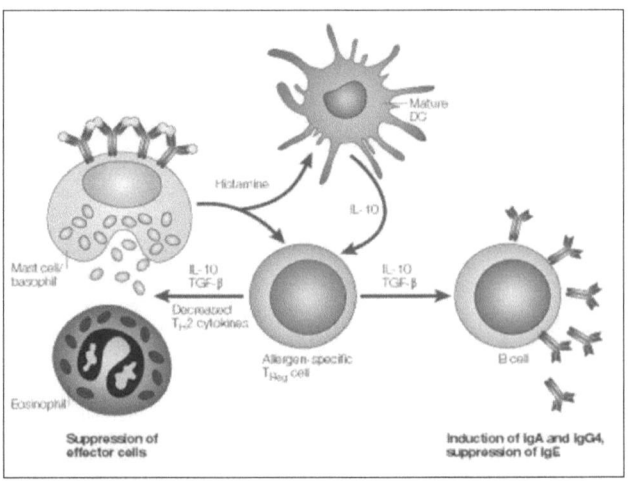

Figure 8: Immune regulation by Treg cells with regard to preventing allergy, taken from Akdis et al, 2003[36]

IL-10 and TGF-β induce tolerogenic antibodies IgG4 and IgA and down-regulate IgE from B cells. These cytokines suppress effector cells of allergy, eg mast cells. The Th2 response is also suppressed through low-level histamine release on their histamine receptor 2.

In allergy, the balance between allergen-specific Treg and Th2 cells is important. Deviation towards a Treg population suppresses Th2 production of pro-inflammatory cytokines, suppresses allergy effector cells, increases IgG4 and IgA production and suppresses IgE[34]. Treg contact-dependent mast cell suppression occurs via the OX40-OX40L interaction. Suppression of Th0/Th1 induction prevents tissue injury mechanisms and IL-10 expression inhibits allergen-induced airway hyperactivity.

Th3 cells are induced by TGF-β and express latency-associated peptide (LAP) on their surface[35]. They express TGF-β and IL-10 and are vital in differentiation of antigen-specific Foxp3+ regulatory cells and maintaining oral tolerance.

Tr1 cells are Foxp3- and require and express IL-10[36]. Their proportion differs between healthy and allergic individuals and they are important mediators in allergy prevention.

Regulatory B cells: Breg, Br1, Br3

These IgM-class cells were recently discovered, characterised by production of inhibitory cytokines including IL-10 and TGF-β. They have different characteristics, mirroring the regulatory T cells (figure 9). Br1 cells produce IL-10, Br3 produces TGF-β and contributes to oral tolerance and Bregs express Foxp3[37]. The tolerogenic effects of these cells include modulation of T cells and inflammation[38], and are important in autoimmunity and allergy. Their absence increases allergy symptoms such as contact hypersensitivity[39].

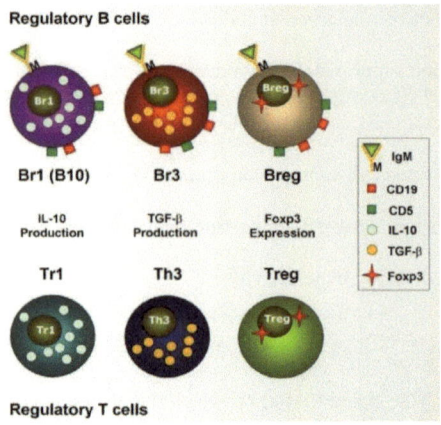

Regulatory B cells

Br1 (B10)   Br3   Breg

IL-10 Production   TGF-β Production   Foxp3 Expression

Tr1   Th3   Treg

Regulatory T cells

IgM
CD19
CD5
IL-10
TGF-β
Foxp3

Figure 9: Overview of the B and T regulatory cells, taken from Noh et al, 2011[39]

The B cell system is similar to the T cell system, with mirrored expression of cytokines and Foxp3.

Innate Immune System: Dendritic cells

DCs induce tolerance with their efficient antigen presenting using MHC and surface proteins[40] and their immunomodulating contact and cytokine mechanisms. DCs are both immunising (figure 5) and tolerogenic (figure 6).

Peripherally, immature DCs constantly sample and present antigens to T cells, but insufficient MHC levels and B7 proteins causes anergy and tolerance[41]. DCs also induce CD8+ tolerance through the PD-1 and CTLA-4 costimulatory mechanisms[42].

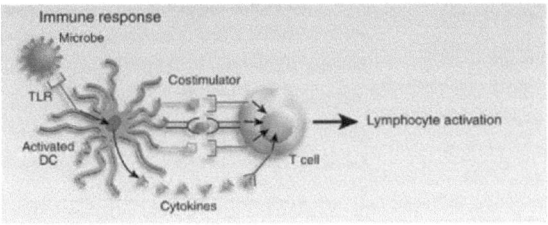

Figure 5: Dendritic cells are capable of activating immune response, modified from Abbas et al, 2005[43]

DCs can be activated in the presence of pathogens and inflammation by Toll-like receptor, leading to NF-κB dependent expression of MHCII, CD40, B7 and proinflammatory cytokines. These function to stimulate lymphocyte activation.

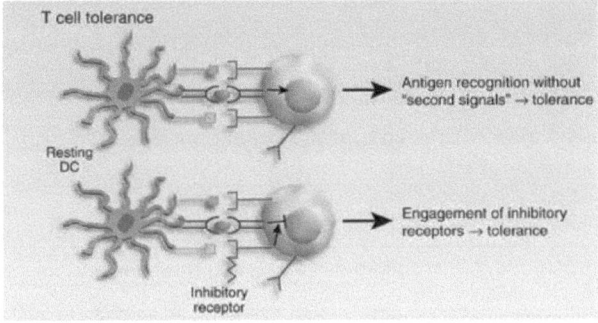

Figure 6: Dendritic cells are capable of tolerance, modified from Abbas et al, 2005[43]

DC can induce anergy in T cells in their naïve state through lack of costimulatory molecules or engagement of inhibitory receptors during antigen presentation.

DCs cause T cell deletion centrally and peripherally, drive the production of Tregs and help polarise Th2 responses[44].

Plasmacytoid DCs (pDCs) are a type 1 IFN-producing sub-type particularly involved in oral tolerance[45] and are found in mucosa, involved in anti-viral and adaptive immune response. They induce tolerance by generating Tregs and Tr1 cells[46] and preventing DTH[47]. Depletion of pDC causes allergic asthma [48] and pulmonary DCs induce Treg development by the ICOS-ICOSL pathway. DCs are therefore necessary in allergy prevention.

Oral Tolerance

Oral tolerance occurs when then gut actively does not respond to foreign antigens when distinguishing between safe and harmful substances. The largest immune organ in the body is the gut associated lymphoid tissue (GALT), primarily Peyer's patches and mesenteric lymph nodes (MLNs)[49]. Peyer's patches contain M-cells which present conventional pathogens to the immune system, whilst MLNs are more important in oral tolerance. Suppression of immune response involves a complex network of non-professional APCs, DCs, Tregs and lymphocytes[50].

Antigen dose affects the tolerance mechanism (table 3), with high dose antigens causing an immediate increase in specific Th1/2 cells, after which surface TCR expression decreases, followed by anergy and then deletion.

Table 3: Relationship between dose of antigen and the mechanisms of oral tolerance induced.

Dose administered	Mechanism of tolerance
High dose	Deletion
	Anergy
	Suppression
Low dose	Th2 cells
	Tr1 cells
	Treg cells

Gut APCs (such as pDC) are conditioned by gut epithelial cells and gut flora, which induces CD103+ retinoic acid-dependent APC that leads to Treg induction at the mucosal surfaces[47]. APCs in the MLNs present antigens to induce a 'founder' population of Tregs, then natural Tregs home to the intestinal lamina propria, where they are expanded and maintained by IL-10-producing CX3CR1$^+$macrophages[51].

Th3 cells are vital in differentiation of antigen-specific Foxp3$^+$Tregs[52]. When Tregs are exposed to antigens they decrease gut autoimmune and inflammatory responses. Anti-CD3 monoclonal antibody is active at mucosal surfaces and induces LAP$^+$ Tregs (TGF-β mediated with elevated Foxp3) which have greater immunosuppressive properties[33].

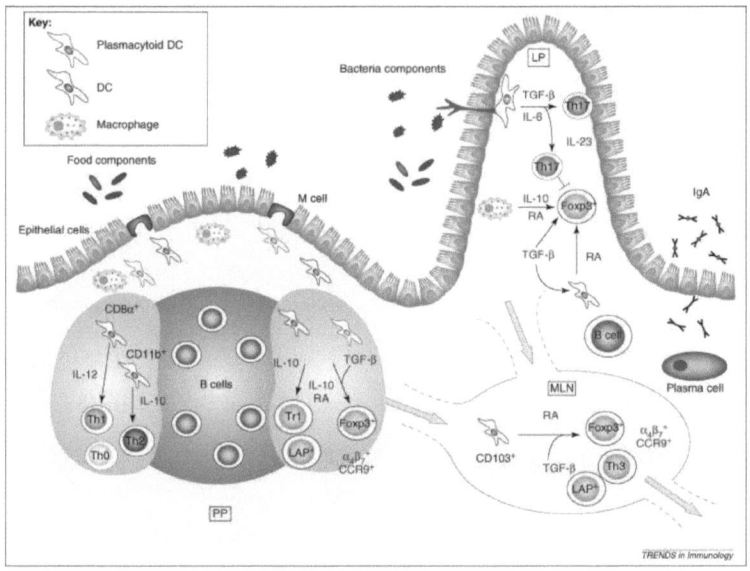

Figure 10: Overview of oral tolerance and T regulatory cell induction, taken from Tsuji et al, 2008[52].

Antigen uptake by M cells and Peyer's patch allows APCs to present to T cells in the GALT or MLN. Retinoic acid from DCs increases Foxp3 expression in T cells, induces LAP+ Tregs and causes IgA class switching in B cells. Foxp3 suppresses T cell function.

Oral tolerance break down can cause hypersensitivities and food allergy[53], with aberrant Treg induction and dysregulated Th2 response causing allergic symptoms.

Immune Privilege

Immune privilege is a form of tolerance generally organ-specific, eg anterior eye chamber, however it can be acquired locally in areas of inflammation through Treg action[54].

Reduced classical MHC with immunoregulatory 1b MHC causes evasion of immune mechanisms[55]. Other factors include local immunosuppressive cytokines such a TGF-β and Fas-FasL dependent apoptosis[56]. This mechanism of tolerance is fairly irrelevant to allergy.

Tolerance in Pregnancy

During pregnancy maternal immune response tolerates the genetically-different foetus and placenta, partly due to immune privilege. HLA-A and –B genes are down-regulated in trophoblast cells and HLA-G class 1b are expressed, protecting from cytotoxic mechanisms[57]. The trophoblast also resists NK- and CTL-mediated lysis.

The immune system undergoes Th2 polarisation, with Tregs causing immunomodulation[58]. Pregnancy also induces foetal antigen-specific maternal Tregs[59]. Pregnancy's effect on maternal allergy has not been explored in great depth, although Th2 deviation could possibly have some effect on atopy.

Induced Tolerance

Where natural tolerance fails to prevent allergy, immunotherapy induces tolerance to specific allergens to alleviate symptoms. Most therapies take advantage of natural tolerance mechanisms. Allergen-specific immunotherapy (allergen-SIT) often induces T cell tolerance and increases Treg, Tr1 and Breg cells and IL-10 production; suppressing pro-inflammatory cells and upregulating non-IgE antibodies (eg IgG4).

Table 4: Describing the different types of allergen-specific immunotherapy

Type of Immunotherapy	Description	Notable Side Effects
Subcutaneous (SCIT)[60, 61]	Tiny doses of allergen injected under the skin gradually increasing until a maintenance dose is reached	Local inflammation and 4% have acute systemic reaction[62]
Intralymphatic (ILIT)[63]	Administer tiny doses of allergen directly to lymph node. Gives quicker better protection with less anaphylaxis	Local discomfort or inflammation
Sublingual (SLIT)[61]	Considered safer but takes longer to reach effectiveness (~3 years)	Local inflammation and exacerbation of autoimmunity
Transcutaneous (TCIT)[64]	Skin patches considered safer and provide effective immunotherapy	Very local inflammation

Oral tolerance can be induced by specific oral tolerance induction (SOTI). In children, successful desensitisation to the allergen occurs over a long period of time[65]. However the side effects, danger of acute reaction and psychological strain make it debatable whether it should be routine practise.

Conclusion

Immunological tolerance is an active process which requires a complex network of different cells and mediators to ensure the body does not mount a harmful response to self and non-self antigens. In allergy, peripheral tolerance is essential to prevent hypersensitivity to innocuous allergens and oral tolerance prevents food allergy. Important factors in maintaining healthy tolerance are T and B cell mechanisms and non-inflammatory cytokines with regulatory cells, as well as DCs, co-ordinating the various components of the immune system. Clinically, immunotherapy is an expanding field which aims to induce tolerance via these mechanisms.

References

(1) Van Parijs L, Abbas AK. Homeostasis and self-tolerance in the immune system: turning lymphocytes off. *Science (New York, N.Y.)* 1998;280(5361): pp. 243-248.

(2) Akdis M. Immune tolerance in allergy. *Current opinion in immunology* 2009;21(6): pp. 700-707.

(3) Akdis CA. Allergy and hypersensitivity: mechanisms of allergic disease. *Current opinion in immunology* 2006;18(6): pp. 718-726.

(4) Romagnani S. Immunologic influences on allergy and the TH1/TH2 balance. *The Journal of allergy and clinical immunology* 2004;113(3): pp. 395-400.

(5) LEDERBERG J. Genes and antibodies. *Science (New York, N.Y.)* 1959;129(3364): pp. 1649-1653.

(6) Smith-Garvin JE, Koretzky GA, Jordan MS. T cell activation. *Annual Review of Immunology* 2009;27: pp. 591-619.

(7) Takahama Y. Journey through the thymus: stromal guides for T-cell development and selection. *Nature reviews.Immunology* 2006;6(2): pp. 127-135.

(8) Haynes BF, Heinly CS. Early human T cell development: analysis of the human thymus at the time of initial entry of hematopoietic stem cells into the fetal thymic microenvironment. *The Journal of experimental medicine* 1995;181(4): pp. 1445-1458.

(9) Mathis D, Benoist C. Aire. *Annual Review of Immunology* 2009;27: pp. 287-312.

(10) Schwartz RH. T cell anergy. *Annual Review of Immunology* 2003;21: pp. 305-334.

(11) Powell JD. The induction and maintenance of T cell anergy. *Clinical immunology (Orlando, Fla.)* 2006;120(3): pp. 239-246.

(12) Appleman LJ, Boussiotis VA. T cell anergy and costimulation. *Immunological reviews* 2003;192: pp. 161-180.

(13) Saeki K, Iwasa Y. T cell anergy as a strategy to reduce the risk of autoimmunity. *Journal of theoretical biology* 2011;277(1): pp. 74-82.

(14) Lim HW, Hillsamer P, Banham AH, Kim CH. Cutting edge: direct suppression of B cells by CD4+ CD25+ regulatory T cells. *Journal of immunology (Baltimore, Md.: 1950)* 2005;175(7): pp. 4180-4183.

(15) Macaubas C, Wahlstrom J, Galvao da Silva AP, Forsthuber TG, Sonderstrup G, Kwok WW, et al. Allergen-specific MHC class II tetramer+ cells are detectable in allergic, but not in nonallergic, individuals. *Journal of immunology (Baltimore, Md.: 1950)* 2006;176(8): pp. 5069-5077.

(16) Marrack P, Kappler J. Control of T cell viability. *Annual Review of Immunology* 2004;22: pp. 765-787.

(17) Chen Y, Inobe J, Marks R, Gonnella P, Kuchroo VK, Weiner HL. Peripheral deletion of antigen-reactive T cells in oral tolerance. *Nature* 1995;376(6536): pp. 177-180.

(18) Stavnezer J, Guikema JE, Schrader CE. Mechanism and regulation of class switch recombination. *Annual Review of Immunology* 2008;26: pp. 261-292.

(19) Wachholz PA, Durham SR. Mechanisms of immunotherapy: IgG revisited. *Current opinion in allergy and clinical immunology* 2004;4(4): pp. 313-318.

(20) Ngoc PL, Gold DR, Tzianabos AO, Weiss ST, Celedon JC. Cytokines, allergy, and asthma. *Current opinion in allergy and clinical immunology* 2005;5(2): pp. 161-166.

(21) Mosmann TR, Coffman RL. TH1 and TH2 cells: different patterns of lymphokine secretion lead to different functional properties. *Annual Review of Immunology* 1989;7: pp. 145-173.

(22) Taylor A, Verhagen J, Blaser K, Akdis M, Akdis CA. Mechanisms of immune suppression by interleukin-10 and transforming growth factor-beta: the role of T regulatory cells. *Immunology* 2006;117(4): pp. 433-442.

(23) Jutel M, Akdis M, Budak F, Aebischer-Casaulta C, Wrzyszcz M, Blaser K, et al. IL-10 and TGF-beta cooperate in the regulatory T cell response to mucosal allergens in normal immunity and specific immunotherapy. *European journal of immunology* 2003;33(5): pp. 1205-1214.

(24) Taylor A, Verhagen J, Akdis CA, Akdis M. T regulatory cells and allergy. *Microbes and Infection* 2005;7(7–8): pp. 1049-1055.

(25) Bour-Jordan H, Esensten JH, Martinez-Llordella M, Penaranda C, Stumpf M, Bluestone JA. Intrinsic and extrinsic control of peripheral T-cell tolerance by costimulatory molecules of the CD28/?B7 family. *Immunological reviews* 2011;241(1): pp. 180-205.

(26) Perez VL, Van Parijs L, Biuckians A, Zheng XX, Strom TB, Abbas AK. Induction of Peripheral T Cell Tolerance In Vivo Requires CTLA-4 Engagement. *Immunity* 1997;6(4): pp. 411-417.

(27) Walunas TL, Lenschow DJ, Bakker CY, Linsley PS, Freeman GJ, Green JM, et al. CTLA-4 can function as a negative regulator of T cell activation. *Immunity* 1994;1(5): pp. 405-413.

(28) Carter L, Fouser LA, Jussif J, Fitz L, Deng B, Wood CR, et al. PD-1:PD-L inhibitory pathway affects both CD4(+) and CD8(+) T cells and is overcome by IL-2. *European journal of immunology* 2002;32(3): pp. 634-643.

(29) Probst HC, McCoy K, Okazaki T, Honjo T, van den Broek M. Resting dendritic cells induce peripheral CD8+ T cell tolerance through PD-1 and CTLA-4. *Nature immunology* 2005;6(3): pp. 280-286.

(30) Umetsu DT, DeKruyff RH. The regulation of allergy and asthma. *Immunological reviews* 2006;212: pp. 238-255.

(31) Jones CA, Holloway JA, Warner JO. Fetal immune responsiveness and routes of allergic sensitization. *Pediatric allergy and immunology : official publication of the European Society of Pediatric Allergy and Immunology* 2002;13 Suppl 15: pp. 19-22.

(32) Gambineri E, Torgerson TR, Ochs HD. Immune dysregulation, polyendocrinopathy, enteropathy, and X-linked inheritance (IPEX), a syndrome of systemic autoimmunity caused by mutations of

FOXP3, a critical regulator of T-cell homeostasis. *Current opinion in rheumatology* 2003;15(4): pp. 430-435.

(33) Shevach EM. Mechanisms of foxp3+ T regulatory cell-mediated suppression. *Immunity* 2009;30(5): pp. 636-645.

(34) Robinson DS, Larche M, Durham SR. Tregs and allergic disease. *The Journal of clinical investigation* 2004;114(10): pp. 1389-1397.

(35) Carrier Y, Yuan J, Kuchroo VK, Weiner HL. Th3 cells in peripheral tolerance. I. Induction of Foxp3-positive regulatory T cells by Th3 cells derived from TGF-beta T cell-transgenic mice. *Journal of immunology (Baltimore, Md.: 1950)* 2007;178(1): pp. 179-185.

(36) Akdis M, Verhagen J, Taylor A, Karamloo F, Karagiannidis C, Crameri R, et al. Immune responses in healthy and allergic individuals are characterized by a fine balance between allergen-specific T regulatory 1 and T helper 2 cells. *The Journal of experimental medicine* 2004;199(11): pp. 1567-1575.

(37) Vitale G, Mion F, Pucillo C. Regulatory B cells: evidence, developmental origin and population diversity. *Molecular immunology* 2010;48(1-3): pp. 1-8.

(38) Lund FE, Randall TD. Effector and regulatory B cells: modulators of CD4(+) T cell immunity. *Nature reviews.Immunology* 2010;10(4): pp. 236-247.

(39) Noh G, Lee JH. Regulatory B cells and allergic diseases. *Allergy, asthma & immunology research* 2011;3(3): pp. 168-177.

(40) Steinman RM. The dendritic cell system and its role in immunogenicity. *Annual Review of Immunology* 1991;9: pp. 271-296.

(41) Steinman RM, Nussenzweig MC. Avoiding horror autotoxicus: the importance of dendritic cells in peripheral T cell tolerance. *Proceedings of the National Academy of Sciences of the United States of America* 2002;99(1): pp. 351-358.

(42) Probst HC, McCoy K, Okazaki T, Honjo T, van den Broek M. Resting dendritic cells induce peripheral CD8+ T cell tolerance through PD-1 and CTLA-4. *Nature immunology* 2005;6(3): pp. 280-286.

(43) Abbas AK, Sharpe AH. Dendritic cells giveth and taketh away. *Nature immunology* 2005;6(3): pp. 227-228.

(44) Hawiger D, Inaba K, Dorsett Y, Guo M, Mahnke K, Rivera M, et al. Dendritic cells induce peripheral T cell unresponsiveness under steady state conditions in vivo. *The Journal of experimental medicine* 2001;194(6): pp. 769-779.

(45) Liu YJ. IPC: professional type 1 interferon-producing cells and plasmacytoid dendritic cell precursors. *Annual Review of Immunology* 2005;23: pp. 275-306.

(46) Wakkach A, Fournier N, Brun V, Breittmayer JP, Cottrez F, Groux H. Characterization of dendritic cells that induce tolerance and T regulatory 1 cell differentiation in vivo. *Immunity* 2003;18(5): pp. 605-617.

(47) Goubier A, Dubois B, Gheit H, Joubert G, Villard-Truc F, Asselin-Paturel C, et al. Plasmacytoid dendritic cells mediate oral tolerance. *Immunity* 2008;29(3): pp. 464-475.

(48) de Heer HJ, Hammad H, Soullie T, Hijdra D, Vos N, Willart MA, et al. Essential role of lung plasmacytoid dendritic cells in preventing asthmatic reactions to harmless inhaled antigen. *The Journal of experimental medicine* 2004;200(1): pp. 89-98.

(49) Weiner HL. Oral tolerance. *Proceedings of the National Academy of Sciences of the United States of America* 1994;91(23): pp. 10762-10765.

(50) Weiner HL. Oral tolerance, an active immunologic process mediated by multiple mechanisms. *The Journal of clinical investigation* 2000;106(8): pp. 935-937.

(51) Hadis U, Wahl B, Schulz O, Hardtke-Wolenski M, Schippers A, Wagner N, et al. Intestinal tolerance requires gut homing and expansion of FoxP3+ regulatory T cells in the lamina propria. *Immunity* 2011;34(2): pp. 237-246.

(52) Tsuji NM, Kosaka A. Oral tolerance: intestinal homeostasis and antigen-specific regulatory T cells. *Trends in immunology* 2008;29(11): pp. 532-540.

(53) Burks AW, Laubach S, Jones SM. Oral tolerance, food allergy, and immunotherapy: Implications for future treatment. *Journal of Allergy and Clinical Immunology* 2008;121(6): pp. 1344-1350.

(54) Cobbold SP, Adams E, Graca L, Daley S, Yates S, Paterson A, et al. Immune privilege induced by regulatory T cells in transplantation tolerance. *Immunological reviews* 2006;213: pp. 239-255.

(55) Niederkorn JY. Mechanisms of immune privilege in the eye and hair follicle. *The journal of investigative dermatology.Symposium proceedings / the Society for Investigative Dermatology, Inc.[and] European Society for Dermatological Research* 2003;8(2): pp. 168-172.

(56) Griffith TS, Brunner T, Fletcher SM, Green DR, Ferguson TA. Fas ligand-induced apoptosis as a mechanism of immune privilege. *Science (New York, N.Y.)* 1995;270(5239): pp. 1189-1192.

(57) Hunt JS, Petroff MG, McIntire RH, Ober C. HLA-G and immune tolerance in pregnancy. *The FASEB journal : official publication of the Federation of American Societies for Experimental Biology* 2005;19(7): pp. 681-693.

(58) Szekeres-Bartho J. Immunological relationship between the mother and the fetus. *International reviews of immunology* 2002;21(6): pp. 471-495.

(59) Kahn DA, Baltimore D. Pregnancy induces a fetal antigen-specific maternal T regulatory cell response that contributes to tolerance. *Proceedings of the National Academy of Sciences of the United States of America* 2010;107(20): pp. 9299-9304.

(60) Burton MJ, Krouse JH, Rosenfeld RM. Extracts from The Cochrane Library: Allergen injection immunotherapy for seasonal allergic rhinitis (review). *Otolaryngology--head and neck surgery : official journal of American Academy of Otolaryngology-Head and Neck Surgery* 2007;136(4): pp. 511-514.

(61) Scadding G, Durham S. Mechanisms of sublingual immunotherapy. *The Journal of asthma : official journal of the Association for the Care of Asthma* 2009;46(4): pp. 322-334.

(62) Bernstein DI, Epstein T, Murphy-Berendts K, Liss GM. Surveillance of systemic reactions to subcutaneous immunotherapy injections: year 1 outcomes of the ACAAI and AAAAI collaborative study. *Annals of Allergy, Asthma & Immunology : Official Publication of the American College of Allergy, Asthma, & Immunology* 2010;104(6): pp. 530-535.

(63) Senti G, Johansen P, Kundig TM. Intralymphatic immunotherapy. *Current opinion in allergy and clinical immunology* 2009;9(6): pp. 537-543.

(64) Senti G, Freiburghaus AU, Kundig TM. Epicutaneous/transcutaneous allergen-specific immunotherapy: rationale and clinical trials. *Current opinion in allergy and clinical immunology* 2010;10(6): pp. 582-586.

(65) Staden U, Rolinck-Werninghaus C, Brewe F, Wahn U, Niggemann B, Beyer K. Specific oral tolerance induction in food allergy in children: efficacy and clinical patterns of reaction. *Allergy* 2007;62(11): pp. 1261-1269.

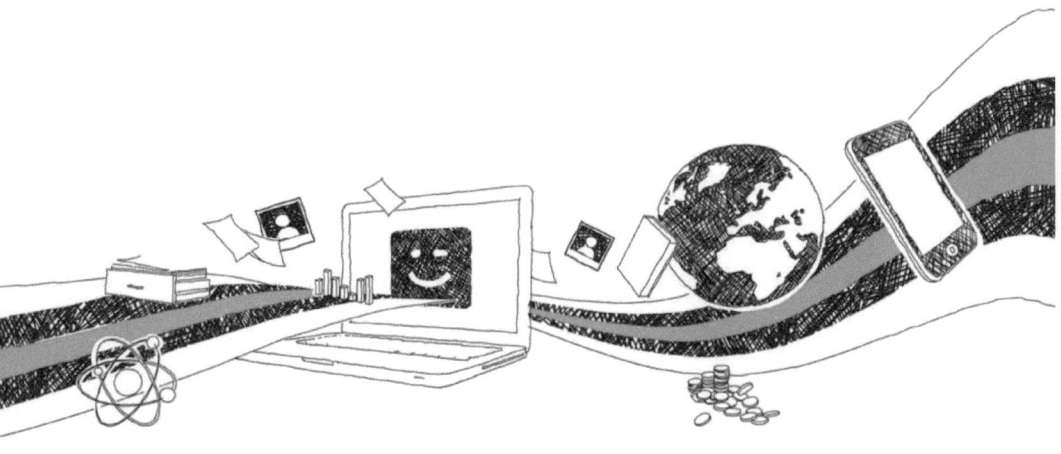
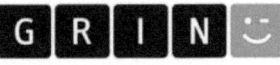